CKD STAGE 3 COOKBOOK FOR SENIORS

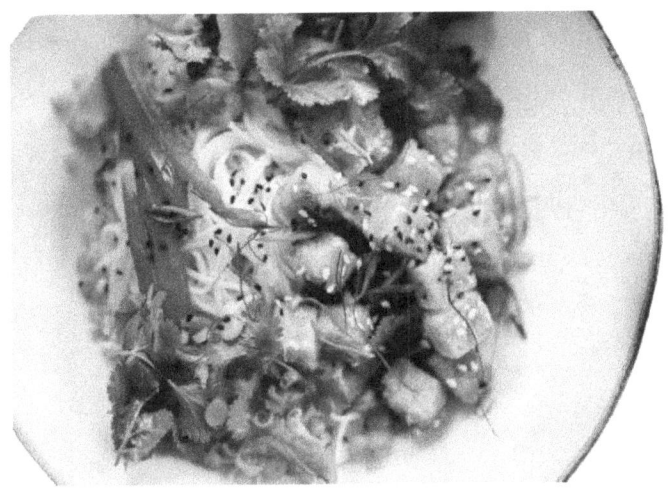

Nutritious Low Potassium, Low Phosphorus,
Low Sodium and Low Protein Recipes

Linda Carlucci

Copyright © 2024 by Linda Carlucci

DISCLAIMER

This cookbook is intended to provide general information and recipes.

The recipes provided in this cookbook are not intended to replace or be a substitute for medical advice from a physician.

The reader should consult a healthcare professional for any specific medical advice, diagnosis or treatment.

Any specific dietary advice provided in this cookbook is not intended to replace or be a substitute for medical advice from a physician.

The author is not responsible or liable for any adverse effects experienced by readers of this cookbook as a result of following the recipes or dietary advice provided.

The author makes no representations or warranties of any kind (express or implied) as to the accuracy, completeness, reliability or suitability of the recipes provided in this cookbook.

The author disclaims any and all liability for any damages arising out of the use or misuse of the recipes provided in this cookbook. The reader must also take care to ensure that the recipes provided in this cookbook are prepared and cooked safely.

The recipes provided in this cookbook are for informational purposes only and should not be used as a substitute for professional medical advice, diagnosis or treatment.

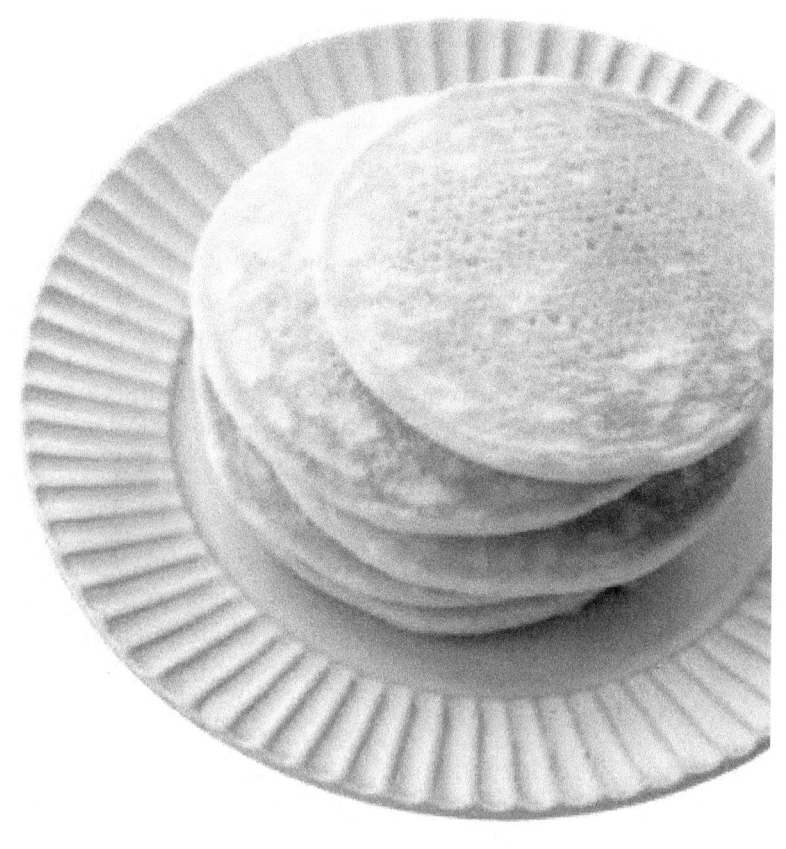

TABLE OF CONTENTS

INTRODUCTION

Chronic Kidney Disease (CKD) stage 3 is characterized by a moderate decrease in kidney function, with a glomerular filtration rate (GFR) of 30-59 ml/min/1.73m².

This stage is crucial as it signifies a significant decline in kidney function and requires close monitoring and management to prevent progression to more severe stages.

The main causes of CKD in seniors include:

- **Diabetes:** Diabetes is one of the leading causes of CKD. High blood sugar levels over time can damage the kidneys' blood vessels and filters, leading to kidney damage.

- **Hypertension:** High blood pressure can damage the kidneys' blood vessels and filters, impairing their ability to function properly.

- **Aging:** As people age, the kidneys naturally undergo changes, such as a decrease in the number of functional nephrons (the kidneys' filtering units), which can contribute to CKD.

- **Glomerulonephritis:** This is a group of diseases that cause inflammation and damage to the kidneys' filtering units (glomeruli), leading to CKD.

- **Polycystic Kidney Disease (PKD):** PKD is a genetic disorder characterized by the growth of cysts in the kidneys, which can lead to CKD over time.

Symptoms of CKD stage 3 in seniors may include:

- Fatigue
- Foamy or bubbly urine
- Increased or decreased urination
- Difficulty concentrating
- Loss of appetite
- Nausea and vomiting
- Itching
- Muscle cramps
- Sleep problems

Early detection and management of CKD stage 3 are crucial to slow down the progression of the disease and reduce the risk of complications. This includes lifestyle modifications (like healthy diet, regular exercise, and quitting smoking).

CHAPTER 1

FOODS TO AVOID FOR CKD STAGE PATIENTS

1. **High-Sodium Foods:** Foods high in sodium can increase blood pressure and worsen fluid retention, leading to swelling and strain on the kidneys. Avoid processed foods, canned soups, and salty snacks.

2. **High-Potassium Foods:** Potassium levels can build up in the blood when kidneys are not functioning properly, leading to dangerous heart rhythm abnormalities. Avoid bananas, oranges, tomatoes, potatoes, and dried fruits.

3. **High-Phosphorus Foods:** High phosphorus levels in the blood can weaken bones and damage blood vessels. Avoid dairy products, nuts, seeds, and whole grains.

4. **High-Protein Foods:** Excessive protein consumption can increase the kidneys' workload and worsen kidney function. Limit intake of meat, poultry, fish, and dairy.

5. **Processed Foods:** Processed foods often contain high levels of sodium, phosphorus, and additives that can be harmful to kidney health. Choose fresh, whole foods instead.

6. **Sugary Foods and Beverages:** High sugar intake can contribute to diabetes and obesity, which are risk factors for CKD progression. Avoid sugary drinks, desserts, and snacks.

7. **Alcohol:** Alcohol can interfere with medications and dehydrate the body, putting additional stress on the kidneys. Limit or avoid alcohol consumption.

8. **Certain Vegetables:** Some vegetables, such as spinach, beet greens, and Swiss chard, are high in potassium and should be consumed in moderation or avoided.

FOODS TO EAT

1. **Low-Potassium Fruits:** Include apples, berries, grapes, and peaches, which are lower in potassium compared to bananas, oranges, and dried fruits. These fruits provide vitamins, minerals, and

antioxidants without raising potassium levels excessively.

2. **Vegetables with Lower Potassium Content:** Go for vegetables like cabbage, carrots, green beans, and onions, which are lower in potassium compared to spinach, potatoes, and tomatoes. These vegetables provide essential nutrients without overloading on potassium.

3. **White Bread and Rice:** Choose white bread and rice over whole grain varieties, as they are lower in phosphorus. This helps reduce phosphorus intake, which is important for kidney health.

4. **Lean Proteins:** Include lean meats like chicken, turkey, and fish in your diet. These proteins are lower in phosphorus and potassium compared to red meats, which can help reduce the strain on the kidneys.

5. **Egg Whites:** Egg whites are a high-quality protein source that is lower in phosphorus and potassium compared to whole eggs. Include egg whites in your diet for protein without the excess phosphorus and potassium.

6. **Low-Dairy or Dairy-Free Alternatives:** Choose low-phosphorus or phosphorus-free dairy alternatives like almond milk or rice milk. These options provide calcium without the phosphorus found in dairy products.

7. **Herbs and Spices:** Use herbs and spices to add flavor to your meals without using salt. This helps reduce sodium intake, which is important for managing blood pressure and fluid balance.

8. **Olive Oil:** Use olive oil as a healthy fat alternative to butter or margarine.

9. **Limited Portions of High-Fiber Foods:** Include limited portions of high-fiber foods like whole grains, fruits, and vegetables to support digestive health, but avoid excessive intake that can be hard on the kidneys.

SALT SUBSTITUTES AND HEALTHY ALTERNATIVES

1. **Herbs and Spices:** Use herbs and spices such as garlic, onion powder, basil, oregano, and black pepper to add flavor to dishes without adding salt.

2. **Vinegar:** Use vinegar, such as balsamic or apple cider vinegar, to add acidity and flavor to meals.

3. **Salt-Free Seasoning Blends:** Look for salt-free seasoning blends that are specifically designed to add flavor without the use of salt.

4. **Herbal Salt Substitutes:** Some products are marketed as salt substitutes and are made from a blend of herbs and spices.

5. **Low-Sodium Soy Sauce:** Use low-sodium soy sauce or tamari as a substitute for regular soy sauce.

6. **Homemade Stocks:** Make your own stocks and broths using fresh ingredients to control the amount of salt added to dishes.

7. **Fresh Herbs and Aromatics:** Use fresh herbs like parsley, cilantro, and dill, as well as aromatics like ginger and garlic, to add flavor to meals.

LIFESTYLE CHANGES FOR EFFECTIVELY MANAGING CKD STAGE FOR SENIORS

1. **Follow a Kidney-Friendly Diet:** Seniors with CKD stage 3 should follow a diet that is low in sodium,

potassium, phosphorus, and protein. This may involve limiting certain foods and beverages and focusing on fresh, whole foods.

2. **Stay Hydrated:** Drinking enough water is important for kidney health. Seniors should aim to drink enough fluids to stay hydrated but not overdo it, especially if they have fluid restrictions.

3. **Monitor Blood Pressure:** High blood pressure can worsen kidney function. Seniors should monitor their blood pressure regularly and work with their healthcare provider to keep it under control.

4. **Manage Blood Sugar Levels:** For seniors with diabetes, keeping blood sugar levels within a healthy range is important for kidney health. This may involve medication, diet, and lifestyle changes.

5. **Stay Active:** Regular physical activity can help improve overall health and manage conditions like high blood pressure and diabetes. Seniors should engage in activities that are safe and appropriate for their fitness level.

6. **Quit Smoking:** Smoking can worsen kidney function and increase the risk of heart disease.

Seniors should quit smoking to improve their overall health.

7. **Limit Alcohol Intake:** Alcohol can interfere with medications and dehydrate the body, putting additional stress on the kidneys. Seniors should limit their alcohol intake or avoid it altogether.

8. **Manage Medications:** Seniors with CKD stage 3 may need to adjust their medications to avoid further damage to the kidneys. It is important to work closely with a healthcare provider to manage medications safely.

9. **Monitor Kidney Function:** Seniors with CKD stage 3 should have regular kidney function tests to monitor the progression of the disease and adjust treatment as needed.

10. **Manage Stress:** Stress can affect overall health and may worsen kidney function. Seniors should find healthy ways to manage stress, such as through relaxation techniques or hobbies.

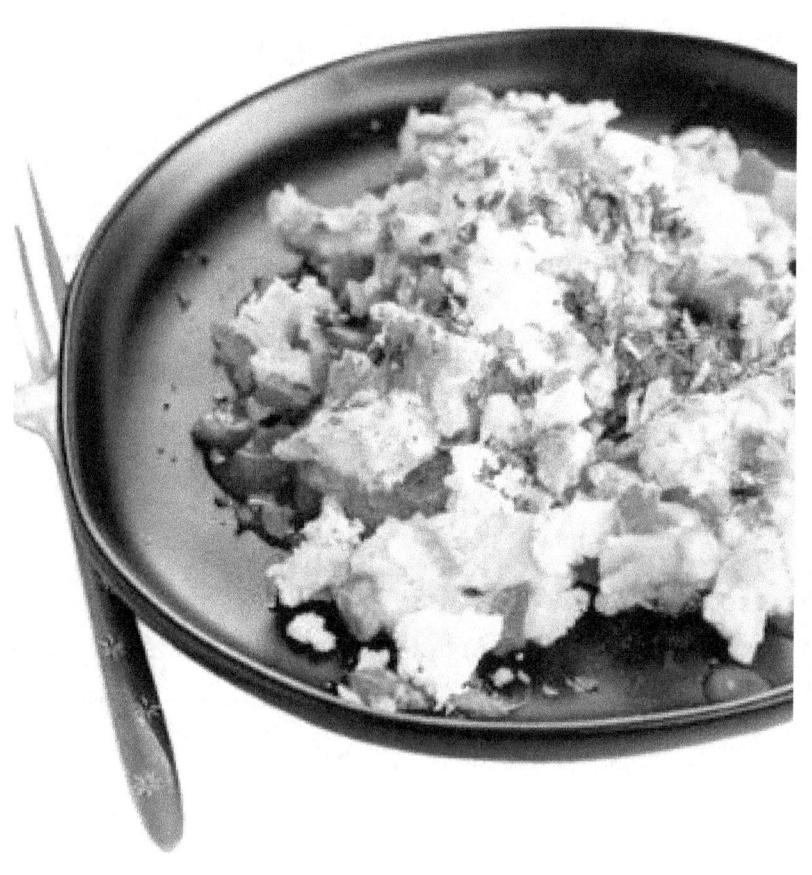

CHAPTER 2

14-DAY MEAL PLAN

DAY 1

Breakfast: Scrambled Eggs with Bell Peppers and Onions

Lunch: Grilled Chicken Salad with Diced Cucumber

Dinner: Greek Salad with Cucumber, Bell Pepper, and Olives

DAY 2

Breakfast: Whole Grain French Toast with Strawberries

Lunch: Turkey Wrap with Lettuce and Bell Pepper

Dinner: Baked Skinless Chicken Breast with Roasted Asparagus

DAY 3

Breakfast: White Rice Porridge with a Sprinkle of Cinnamon and Sliced Peaches

Lunch: Cauliflower Stir-Fry with Tofu

Dinner: Grilled Salmon with Sautéed Lettuce and White Rice

DAY 4

Breakfast: White Rice Flour Pancakes with Blueberries

Lunch: Baked Salmon with Steamed Broccoli

Dinner: Turkey Meatballs with Zucchini Noodles and Bell Pepper Sauce

DAY 5

Breakfast: Smoothie made with Berries and Apple Juice

Lunch: Turkey Chili made with Lean Ground Turkey and Bell Pepper

Dinner: Stir-Fried Tofu with Broccoli and Bell Peppers

DAY 6

Breakfast: Whole Grain Bread Toast with a Small Amount of Margarine and Sugar-Free Jelly

Lunch: Egg Salad Sandwich on Whole Grain Bread with Lettuce and Bell Pepper

Dinner: Baked Cod with Steamed Green Beans and a Side Salad

DAY 7

Breakfast: Breakfast Burrito with Scrambled Eggs, Swiss Cheese, and Salsa

Lunch: Veggie Burger on a Whole Grain Bun with Lettuce and Cabbage

Dinner: Chicken and Vegetable Kebabs Served with Couscous

DAY 8

Lunch: Tuna Salad with Celery and Onion on Whole Grain Crackers

Breakfast: White Rice Cake with a Drizzle of Natural Sweetener

Dinner: Cauliflower Curry with Green Beans Served Over Bulgur Rice

DAY 9

Lunch: Boiled Corn Salad with Bell Peppers, Red Onion, and Celery

Breakfast: Cauliflower Omelet made with Bell Peppers

Dinner: Shrimp Stir-Fry with Mixed Lettuce and Bell Pepper

DAY 10

Lunch: Grilled Chicken Breast with Steamed Green Beans

Breakfast: Whole Wheat Muffin with a Side of Grapes

Dinner: Stuffed Bell Peppers with Ground Turkey and Diced Bell Pepper

DAY 11

Breakfast: Scrambled Eggs with Bell Peppers and Onions

Lunch: Grilled Chicken Salad with Diced Cucumber

Dinner: Greek Salad with Cucumber, Bell Pepper, and Olives

DAY 12

Breakfast: Whole Grain French Toast with Strawberries

Lunch: Turkey Wrap with Lettuce and Bell Pepper

Dinner: Baked Skinless Chicken Breast with Roasted Asparagus

DAY 13

Breakfast: White Rice Porridge with a Sprinkle of Cinnamon and Sliced Peaches

Lunch: Cauliflower Stir-Fry with Tofu

Dinner: Grilled Salmon with Sautéed Lettuce and White Rice

DAY 14

Breakfast: White Rice Flour Pancakes with Blueberries

Lunch: Baked Salmon with Steamed Broccoli

Dinner: Turkey Meatballs with Zucchini Noodles and Bell Pepper Sauce

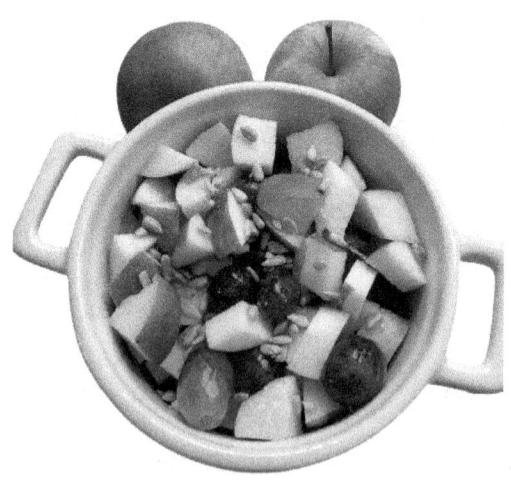

CHAPTER 3

NUTRITIOUS RECIPES FOR A CKD STAGE 3 DIET FOR SENIORS

BREAKFAST

Scrambled Eggs with Bell Peppers and Onions

Preparation Time: 10 minutes

Serves: 2

Calories: 150 **Potassium:** 40mg **Phosphorus:** 40mg **Sodium:** 35mg

Ingredients:

4 large eggs

1/4 cup chopped bell peppers (choose red or yellow for lower potassium)

1/4 cup chopped onions

1 tablespoon olive oil

A pinch of salt and pepper

Method of Preparation:

1. Heat olive oil in a non-stick skillet over medium heat.
2. Add chopped bell peppers and onions to the skillet and sauté until softened, about 3-4 minutes.
3. In a bowl, whisk the eggs with salt and pepper.
4. Pour the eggs into the skillet with the bell peppers and onions.
5. Cook, stirring occasionally, until the eggs are scrambled and cooked to your desired consistency.
6. Serve hot, garnished with a sprinkle of chopped parsley if desired.

Whole Grain French Toast with Strawberries

Preparation Time: 15 minutes

Serves: 2

Calories: 220 **Potassium:** 40mg **Phosphorus:** 50mg **Sodium:** 40mg

Ingredients:

4 slices of whole grain bread (low sodium)

2 large eggs

1/4 cup low-fat milk

1/2 teaspoon vanilla extract

1/2 teaspoon ground cinnamon

Cooking spray

Fresh strawberries for topping (optional)

Method of Preparation:

1. In a shallow bowl, whisk together eggs, milk, vanilla extract, and ground cinnamon.
2. Heat a non-stick skillet or griddle over medium heat and lightly coat with cooking spray.
3. Dip each slice of bread into the egg mixture, ensuring both sides are coated evenly.
4. Place the dipped bread slices onto the skillet and cook until golden brown on both sides, about 2-3 minutes per side.
5. Serve hot, topped with fresh strawberries if desired.

White Rice Porridge with a Sprinkle of Cinnamon and Sliced Peaches

Preparation Time: 25 minutes

Serves: 2

Calories: 200 **Potassium:** 30mg **Phosphorus:** 50mg **Sodium:** 0mg

Ingredients:

1/2 cup white rice

2 cups water

1/2 teaspoon ground cinnamon

1 medium peach, sliced

Method of Preparation:

1. Rinse the white rice under cold water until the water runs clear.
2. In a pot, bring 2 cups of water to a boil.
3. Add the rinsed rice to the boiling water, reduce heat to low, and cover.

4. Simmer the rice for 15-20 minutes, or until the rice is cooked and the water is absorbed, stirring occasionally.

5. Once the rice is cooked, sprinkle ground cinnamon over the porridge and stir to combine.

6. Serve hot, topped with sliced peaches.

White Rice Flour Pancakes with Blueberries

Preparation Time: 20 minutes

Serves: 2

Calories: 250 **Potassium:** 40mg **Phosphorus:** 40mg

Ingredients:

1 cup white rice flour

1 tablespoon baking powder (low-sodium)

1 tablespoon sugar substitute

1 cup unsweetened almond milk

2 tablespoons vegetable oil

1/2 teaspoon vanilla extract

1/2 cup fresh blueberries

Method of Preparation:

1. In a mixing bowl, combine the white rice flour, baking powder, and sugar substitute.
2. Add the almond milk, vegetable oil, and vanilla extract to the dry ingredients.
3. Mix until just combined.
4. Gently fold in the blueberries.
5. Heat a non-stick skillet or griddle over medium heat and lightly grease with vegetable oil or cooking spray.
6. Pour 1/4 cup of batter onto the skillet for each pancake.
7. Cook until bubbles form on the surface of the pancake, then flip and cook until golden brown on both sides.
8. Serve warm with additional blueberries on top if desired.

Smoothie made with Berries and Apple Juice

Preparation Time: 5 minutes

Serves: 1

Calories: 70 **Potassium:** 50mg **Phosphorus:** 30mg

Ingredients:

1/2 cup mixed berries (such as strawberries, raspberries, and blueberries)

1/2 cup unsweetened apple juice

1/2 cup ice cubes

1/4 cup plain Greek yogurt (low-phosphorus)

Method of Preparation:

1. Place the mixed berries, apple juice, ice cubes, and Greek yogurt in a blender.
2. Blend until smooth and creamy.
3. Pour into glasses and serve immediately.

Whole Grain Bread Toast with a Small Amount of Margarine and Sugar-Free Jelly

Preparation Time: 5 minutes

Serves: 2

Calories: 150 **Potassium:** 30mg **Phosphorus:** 40mg

Ingredients:

4 slices whole grain bread (low-sodium)

2 teaspoons margarine (low-sodium)

Sugar-free jelly (choose a variety low in phosphorus)

Method of Preparation:

1. Toast the whole grain bread slices until golden brown.
2. Spread 1/2 teaspoon of margarine on each slice of toast.
3. Top with a small amount of sugar-free jelly.

Breakfast Burrito with Scrambled Eggs, Swiss Cheese, and Salsa

Preparation Time: 15 minutes

Serves: 2

Calories: 340 **Potassium:** 25mg **Phosphorus:** 45mg

Ingredients:

4 large eggs

1/4 cup shredded Swiss cheese

4 whole wheat tortillas (low-sodium if available)

1/2 cup low-sodium salsa

Cooking spray (or olive oil spray)

Note: Omit salt or use a low-sodium substitute.

Method of Preparation:

1. Crack the eggs into a bowl and beat them until well combined.
2. Heat a non-stick skillet over medium heat and lightly coat with cooking spray.

3. Pour the beaten eggs into the skillet and cook, stirring occasionally, until scrambled and fully cooked.

4. Divide the scrambled eggs evenly among the tortillas.

5. Sprinkle each portion with 1 tablespoon of shredded Swiss cheese.

6. Roll up the tortillas, folding in the ends to enclose the filling.

7. Serve the breakfast burritos with low-sodium salsa on the side.

White Rice Cake with a Drizzle of Natural Sweetener

Preparation Time: 2 minutes

Serves: 2

Calories: 70 **Potassium:** 10mg **Phosphorus:** 20mg

Ingredients:

2 white rice cakes

1 tablespoon natural sweetener (such as honey or maple syrup)

Cinnamon (optional)

Method of Preparation:

1. Place the white rice cakes on a serving plate.
2. Drizzle 1/2 tablespoon of natural sweetener over each rice cake.
3. Sprinkle with cinnamon, if desired.

Cauliflower Omelet made with Bell Peppers

Preparation Time: 15 minutes

Serves: 2

Calories: 150 **Potassium:** 40mg **Phosphorus:** 60mg

Ingredients:

1 cup cauliflower florets (unsuitable, replace with zucchini)

1/2 red bell pepper, diced

1/2 green bell pepper, diced

4 eggs

2 tablespoons low-fat milk (unsuitable, replace with unsweetened almond milk)

A pinch of salt and pepper

1 tablespoon olive oil

Method of Preparation:

1. Heat olive oil in a non-stick skillet over medium heat.
2. Add diced bell peppers to the skillet and sauté until slightly softened, about 3-4 minutes.
3. In a bowl, whisk together eggs, unsweetened almond milk, salt, and pepper.
4. Pour the egg mixture over the sautéed bell peppers in the skillet.
5. Cook until the edges of the omelet begin to set, then gently lift the edges with a spatula to let the uncooked eggs flow underneath.
6. Once the omelet is mostly set, sprinkle the top with diced zucchini.
7. Carefully fold the omelet in half and cook for another 1-2 minutes until cooked through.
8. Slide the omelet onto a plate and serve warm.

Whole Wheat Muffin with a Side of Grapes

Preparation Time: 10 minutes

Serves: 2

Calories: 180 **Potassium:** 45mg **Phosphorus:** 40mg

Ingredients:

2 whole wheat muffins

1 cup grapes

Method of Preparation:

1. Preheat the oven to 350°F (175°C).
2. Place the whole wheat muffins on a baking sheet and warm them in the oven for 5-7 minutes.
3. Wash the grapes thoroughly under running water and pat them dry.
4. Serve the warm whole wheat muffins with a side of fresh grapes.

LUNCH

Grilled Chicken Salad with Diced Cucumber

Preparation Time: 20 minutes

Serves: 2

Calories: 250 **Potassium:** 40mg **Phosphorus:** 45mg

Ingredients:

2 boneless, skinless chicken breasts

2 cups diced cucumber

4 cups mixed salad greens

1 tablespoon olive oil

1 tablespoon lemon juice

A pinch of salt and pepper

Method of Preparation:

1. Preheat grill to medium-high heat.
2. Season chicken breasts with salt, pepper, and olive oil.

3. Grill chicken breasts for 6-8 minutes per side, or until cooked through.

4. Remove chicken from grill and let it rest for 5 minutes before slicing.

5. In a large bowl, combine diced cucumber and mixed salad greens.

6. In a small bowl, whisk together olive oil, lemon juice, salt, and pepper to make the dressing.

7. Add sliced grilled chicken to the salad mixture.

8. Drizzle dressing over the salad and toss gently to coat.

9. Divide the salad into 2 servings and serve immediately.

Turkey Wrap with Lettuce and Bell Pepper

Preparation Time: 15 minutes

Serves: 2

Calories: 220 **Potassium:** 30mg **Phosphorus:** 40mg

Ingredients:

4 slices low-sodium turkey breast

4 large lettuce leaves

1 bell pepper, thinly sliced

4 tablespoons hummus (low-sodium)

2 whole grain tortillas

Method of Preparation:

1. Lay out the tortillas and spread 2 tablespoons of hummus evenly over each tortilla.
2. Place 2 slices of turkey breast on each tortilla.
3. Top with lettuce leaves and thinly sliced bell pepper.
4. Roll up the tortillas tightly.
5. Cut each wrap in half and serve.

Cauliflower Stir-Fry with Tofu

Preparation Time: 25 minutes

Serves: 2

Calories: 180 **Potassium:** 45mg **Phosphorus:** 35mg

Ingredients:

1 head cauliflower, cut into florets

200g firm tofu, cubed

1 bell pepper, sliced

1 cup sliced mushrooms

2 cloves garlic, minced

2 tablespoons low-sodium soy sauce

1 tablespoon olive oil

1 teaspoon grated ginger

Sesame seeds for garnish (optional)

Method of Preparation:

1. Heat olive oil in a large skillet over medium heat.

2. Add minced garlic and grated ginger to the skillet and sauté for 1-2 minutes.

3. Add cauliflower florets, sliced bell pepper, and sliced mushrooms to the skillet.

4. Cook for 5-7 minutes, stirring occasionally, until vegetables are tender.

5. Push vegetables to one side of the skillet and add cubed tofu to the empty space.

6. Cook tofu for 3-4 minutes, or until lightly browned.

7. Stir tofu into the vegetable mixture.

8. Pour soy sauce over the stir-fry and toss to coat evenly.

9. Garnish with sesame seeds if desired and serve hot.

Baked Salmon with Steamed Broccoli

Preparation Time: 20 minutes

Serves: 2

Calories: 300 **Potassium:** 300 mg **Phosphorus:** 50 mg

Ingredients:

2 salmon fillets (about 4 oz each)

2 cups broccoli florets

2 teaspoons olive oil

1/4 teaspoon garlic powder

1/4 teaspoon lemon pepper

1/4 teaspoon dried dill

A pinch of salt and pepper

Method of Preparation:

1. Preheat your oven to 375°F (190°C).

2. Place the salmon fillets on a baking sheet lined with parchment paper.

3. Drizzle each fillet with 1 teaspoon of olive oil, then sprinkle with garlic powder, lemon pepper, dried dill, salt, and pepper.

4. Bake in the preheated oven for 12-15 minutes, or until the salmon is cooked through and flakes easily with a fork.

5. While the salmon is baking, steam the broccoli florets until tender, about 5-7 minutes.

6. Serve the baked salmon with steamed broccoli on the side.

Turkey Chili made with Lean Ground Turkey and Bell Peppers

Preparation Time: 35 minutes

Serves: 2

Calories: 350 **Potassium:** 60 mg **Phosphorus:** 60 mg

Ingredients:

1 lb. lean ground turkey

1 onion, diced

2 cloves garlic, minced

1 bell pepper, diced (use a low-potassium variety such as red or yellow)

1 teaspoon ground cumin

1 teaspoon chili powder

A pinch of salt and pepper

Chopped fresh cilantro for garnish (optional)

Method of Preparation:

1. In a large pot, brown the ground turkey over medium heat until cooked through.
2. Add the diced onion, minced garlic, and diced bell pepper to the pot, and cook until softened, about 5 minutes.
3. Stir in the ground cumin, chili powder, salt, and pepper.

4. Simmer the chili uncovered for 20-25 minutes, stirring occasionally, until flavors are well combined.

5. Serve the turkey chili hot, garnished with chopped fresh cilantro if desired.

Egg Salad Sandwich on Whole Grain Bread with Lettuce and Bell Peppers

Preparation Time: 15 minutes

Serves: 2

Calories: 300 **Potassium:** 50 mg **Phosphorus:** 70 mg

Ingredients:

4 hard-boiled eggs, chopped

2 tablespoons low-fat mayonnaise

1 tablespoon Dijon mustard

1 stalk celery, finely chopped

1 bell pepper, diced (use a low-potassium variety such as red or yellow)

4 slices whole grain bread

Lettuce leaves for topping

Method of Preparation:

1. In a mixing bowl, combine the chopped hard-boiled eggs, low-fat mayonnaise, Dijon mustard, and finely chopped celery. Stir until well combined.
2. Place the diced bell pepper into the egg mixture and stir to incorporate.
3. Toast the whole grain bread slices until lightly golden.
4. Divide the egg salad mixture evenly between two slices of toasted bread.
5. Top each with lettuce leaves and the remaining slices of toasted bread.
6. Cut each sandwich in half and serve.

Veggie Burger on a Whole Grain Buns with Lettuce and Cabbage

Preparation Time: 15 minutes

Serves: 2

Calories: 350 **Potassium:** 40mg **Phosphorus:** 45mg
Sodium: 18mg

Ingredients:

2 whole grain burger buns

2 veggie burger patties

2 lettuce leaves

1 cup shredded cabbage

1 tablespoon olive oil

A pinch of salt and pepper

Method of Preparation:

1. Heat olive oil in a pan over medium heat.
2. Cook veggie burger patties for 3-4 minutes on each side until golden brown.
3. Toast whole grain buns until lightly crispy.
4. Place lettuce leaves on the bottom half of each bun.
5. Put the cooked veggie burger patties on top of the lettuce.
6. Add shredded cabbage on top of the patties.
7. Season with A pinch of salt and pepper.
8. Cover with the top half of the bun.
9. Serve warm.

Tuna Salad with Celery and Onion on Whole Grain Crackers

Preparation Time: 10 minutes

Serves: 2

Calories: 220 **Potassium:** 45mg **Phosphorus:** 40mg **Sodium:** 15mg

Ingredients:

1 can (5 ounces) low-sodium tuna, drained

1 stalk celery, finely chopped

1/4 onion, finely chopped

2 tablespoons plain Greek yogurt

1 tablespoon lemon juice

A pinch of salt and pepper

Whole Grain Crackers:

8 whole grain crackers

Method of Preparation:

1. In a bowl, combine drained tuna, chopped celery, chopped onion, Greek yogurt, and lemon juice.
2. Mix well until all ingredients are evenly combined.
3. Season with A pinch of salt and pepper.
4. Spoon tuna salad onto whole grain crackers.
5. Serve immediately.

Boiled Corn Salad with Bell Peppers and Red Onion

Preparation Time: 15 minutes

Serves: 2

Calories: 120 **Potassium:** 45mg **Phosphorus:** 30mg

Ingredients:

2 ears of corn, husked and kernels removed

1 red bell pepper, diced

1/2 red onion, finely chopped

2 tablespoons fresh parsley, chopped

1 tablespoon olive oil

1 tablespoon lemon juice

A pinch of salt and pepper

Method of Preparation:

1. Bring a pot of water to a boil.
2. Add the corn kernels and cook for 3-4 minutes until tender.
3. Drain and let cool.
4. In a large mixing bowl, combine the boiled corn kernels, diced red bell pepper, chopped red onion, diced celery, and chopped parsley.
5. In a small bowl, whisk together the olive oil and lemon juice. Pour the dressing over the salad mixture and toss to coat evenly.
6. Season with A pinch of salt and pepper.
7. Serve immediately or refrigerate until ready to serve.

Grilled Chicken Breast with Steamed Green Beans

Preparation Time: 20 minutes

Serves: 2

Calories: 200 **Potassium:** 40mg **Phosphorus:** 40mg

Ingredients:

2 boneless, skinless chicken breasts

1/2 teaspoon rosemary powder

1/2 teaspoon thyme powder

A pinch of salt and pepper

1 tablespoon olive oil

1 cup green beans, trimmed

Lemon wedges for serving (optional)

Method of Preparation:

1. Preheat grill to medium-high heat.
2. Season the chicken breasts with garlic powder, onion powder, salt, and pepper.
3. Drizzle olive oil over the chicken breasts and rub to coat evenly.
4. Grill the chicken breasts for 6-8 minutes per side, or until cooked through and no longer pink in the center.
5. Remove from grill and let rest for a few minutes.

6. Meanwhile, steam the green beans until tender, about 4-5 minutes.

7. Serve the grilled chicken breasts with steamed green beans on the side.

8. Squeeze lemon wedges over the chicken for added flavor, if desired.

DINNER

Greek Salad with Cucumber, Bell Pepper, and Olives

Preparation Time: 15 minutes

Serves: 2

Calories: 180 **Potassium:** 60mg **Phosphorus:** 40mg **Sodium:** 150mg

Ingredients:

2 medium cucumbers, peeled and diced

1 red bell pepper, diced

1 yellow bell pepper, diced

1/2 red onion, thinly sliced

1/2 cup Kalamata olives, pitted and sliced

2 tablespoons extra virgin olive oil

2 tablespoons red wine vinegar

1 teaspoon dried oregano

A pinch of salt and pepper

1/4 cup crumbled feta cheese (optional, for garnish)

Method of Preparation:

1. In a large bowl, combine the cucumbers, bell peppers, red onion, and olives.
2. In a small bowl, whisk together the olive oil, red wine vinegar, dried oregano, salt, and pepper.
3. Pour the dressing over the salad and toss to coat evenly.
4. Divide the salad between two plates and garnish with crumbled feta cheese if desired.

Baked Skinless Chicken Breast with Roasted Asparagus

Preparation Time: 30 minutes

Serves: 2

Calories: 280 **Potassium:** 50mg **Phosphorus:** 45mg **Sodium:** 40mg

Ingredients:

2 skinless chicken breasts

1 bunch asparagus, trimmed

2 tablespoons olive oil

2 cloves garlic, minced

1 teaspoon dried thyme

A pinch of salt and pepper

Lemon wedges for serving

Method of Preparation:

1. Preheat your oven to 400°F (200°C).
2. Place the chicken breasts on a baking sheet lined with parchment paper.
3. Arrange the asparagus around the chicken on the baking sheet.

4. In a small bowl, whisk together the olive oil, minced garlic, dried thyme, salt, and pepper.

5. Drizzle the olive oil mixture over the chicken and asparagus, making sure everything is evenly coated.

6. Bake in the preheated oven for 20-25 minutes, or until the chicken is cooked through and the asparagus is tender.

7. Serve the chicken and asparagus with lemon wedges on the side.

Grilled Salmon with Sautéed Lettuce and White Rice

Preparation Time: 25 minutes

Serves: 2

Calories: 320 **Potassium:** 40mg **Phosphorus:** 50mg **Sodium:** 15mg

Ingredients:

2 salmon fillets

1 tablespoon olive oil

1 teaspoon lemon juice

A pinch of salt and pepper

1 head iceberg lettuce, chopped

1 tablespoon unsalted butter

1 cup cooked white rice

Method of Preparation:

1. Preheat your grill to medium-high heat.
2. In a small bowl, mix together the olive oil, lemon juice, salt, and pepper.
3. Brush the mixture over the salmon fillets.
4. Grill the salmon fillets for 4-5 minutes per side, or until cooked to your desired doneness.
5. In a skillet, melt the butter over medium heat.
6. Add the chopped lettuce and sauté for 2-3 minutes, or until wilted.
7. Serve the grilled salmon alongside the sautéed lettuce and cooked white rice.

Turkey Meatballs with Zucchini Noodles and Bell Pepper Sauce

Preparation Time: 35 minutes

Serves: 2

Calories: 320 **Potassium:** 420 mg **Phosphorus:** 40 mg **Sodium:** 15 mg

Ingredients:

1 lb. lean ground turkey

2 medium zucchinis, spiralized into noodles

1 red bell pepper, diced

1 yellow bell pepper, diced

1 onion, diced

2 cloves garlic, minced

1 tablespoon olive oil

1 tablespoon chopped fresh basil

A pinch of salt and pepper

For the Bell Pepper Sauce:

2 red bell peppers, roasted and peeled

1 clove garlic

2 tablespoons olive oil

A pinch of salt and pepper

Method of Preparation:

1. Preheat the oven to 375°F (190°C).

2. In a large bowl, combine the ground turkey, diced onions, minced garlic, chopped basil, salt, and pepper.

3. Mix well and shape the mixture into meatballs.

4. Place the meatballs on a baking sheet lined with parchment paper and bake for 20-25 minutes or until cooked through.

5. While the meatballs are baking, prepare the bell pepper sauce. In a blender, combine the roasted red bell peppers, garlic, olive oil, salt, and pepper.

6. Blend until smooth.

7. Heat olive oil in a skillet over medium heat.

8. Add diced bell peppers and sauté until tender.

9. Add the zucchini noodles to the skillet and cook for 2-3 minutes until heated through but still crisp.

10. Serve the turkey meatballs over the zucchini noodles and bell pepper sauce.

Stir-Fried Tofu with Broccoli and Bell Peppers

Preparation Time: 25 minutes

Serves: 2

Calories: 280 **Potassium:** 80 mg **Phosphorus:** 50 mg **Sodium:** 30 mg

Ingredients:

14 oz firm tofu, drained and cubed

2 cups broccoli florets

1 red bell pepper, sliced

1 yellow bell pepper, sliced

2 cloves garlic, minced

2 tablespoons low-sodium soy sauce

1 tablespoon sesame oil

1 tablespoon rice vinegar

1 teaspoon grated ginger

1 tablespoon olive oil

Method of Preparation:

1. Heat olive oil in a large skillet over medium heat.
2. Add minced garlic and grated ginger, and sauté for 1 minute.
3. Add cubed tofu to the skillet and stir-fry until golden brown.
4. Add broccoli florets and sliced bell peppers to the skillet.
5. Stir-fry for 3-4 minutes until vegetables are tender-crisp.
6. In a small bowl, whisk together low-sodium soy sauce, sesame oil, and rice vinegar.
7. Pour the sauce over the tofu and vegetables, and stir to combine.
8. Cook for an additional 2 minutes, then remove from heat.
9. Serve hot.

Baked Cod with Steamed Green Beans and a Side Salad

Preparation Time: 30 minutes

Serves: 2

Calories: 320 **Potassium:** 70 mg **Phosphorus:** 45 mg **Sodium:** 10 mg

Ingredients:

2 cod fillets (about 6 oz each)

2 cups green beans, trimmed

2 cups mixed salad greens

1 tomato, sliced

1 cucumber, sliced

2 tablespoons olive oil

1 tablespoon lemon juice

1 teaspoon dried dill

A pinch of salt and pepper

Method of Preparation:

1. Preheat the oven to 375°F (190°C).

2. Place the cod fillets on a baking sheet lined with parchment paper.

3. Drizzle with olive oil and lemon juice, then sprinkle with dried dill, salt, and pepper.

4. Bake for 15-20 minutes, or until the fish is cooked through and flakes easily with a fork.

5. While the cod is baking, steam the green beans until tender.

6. Assemble the salad by combining mixed salad greens, sliced tomato, and cucumber in a bowl.

7. Drizzle the salad with olive oil and lemon juice, and season with A pinch of salt and pepper.

8. Serve the baked cod with steamed green beans and a side salad.

Chicken and Vegetable Kebabs Served with Couscous

Preparation Time: 20 minutes

Serves: 2

Calories: 380 **Potassium:** 45mg **Phosphorus:** 40mg

Ingredients:

2 boneless, skinless chicken breasts, cut into cubes

1 red bell pepper, cut into chunks

1 green bell pepper, cut into chunks

1 small red onion, cut into chunks

2 tablespoons olive oil

1 teaspoon dried oregano

1 teaspoon paprika

1/2 teaspoon garlic powder

A pinch of salt and pepper

1 cup couscous

1 1/4 cups low-sodium chicken broth

Method of Preparation:

1. Preheat your grill to medium-high heat.
2. In a bowl, combine the cubed chicken, bell peppers, onion, olive oil, oregano, paprika, garlic powder, salt, and pepper.
3. Toss until everything is evenly coated.
4. Thread the marinated chicken and vegetables onto skewers.

5. Grill the kebabs for 10-12 minutes, turning occasionally, until the chicken is cooked through and the vegetables are tender.

6. While the kebabs are grilling, prepare the couscous according to the package instructions, using low-sodium chicken broth instead of water.

7. Serve the grilled chicken and vegetable kebabs with the cooked couscous.

Cauliflower Curry with Green Beans Served Over Bulgur Rice

Preparation Time: 30 minutes

Serves: 2

Calories: 320 **Potassium:** 40mg **Phosphorus:** 45mg

Ingredients:

1 small head cauliflower, cut into florets

1 cup green beans, trimmed and cut into bite-sized pieces

1 tablespoon olive oil

1 small onion, finely chopped

2 cloves garlic, minced

1 tablespoon curry powder

1 teaspoon ground turmeric

1/2 teaspoon ground cumin

1/2 teaspoon ground coriander

1/4 teaspoon cayenne pepper (optional)

1/2 cup low-sodium vegetable broth

A pinch of salt and pepper

1 cup bulgur rice

1 1/4 cups water

Method of Preparation:

1. Heat the olive oil in a large skillet over medium heat.
2. Add the onion and garlic, and cook until softened, about 3-4 minutes.
3. Add the cauliflower florets to the skillet and cook for 5 minutes, stirring occasionally.

4. Stir in the curry powder, turmeric, cumin, coriander, and cayenne pepper (if using), and cook for an additional 2 minutes.

5. Pour in the vegetable broth, and bring to a simmer.

6. Cook for 10-12 minutes, or until the cauliflower is tender.

7. While the cauliflower curry is cooking, prepare the bulgur rice.

8. In a separate saucepan, bring the water to a boil.

9. Stir in the bulgur rice, cover, and remove from heat.

10. Let it sit for 10 minutes, then fluff with a fork.

11. Add the green beans to the cauliflower curry and cook for an additional 3-4 minutes, until the green beans are tender-crisp.

12. Serve the cauliflower curry over the bulgur rice.

Shrimp Stir-Fry with Mixed Lettuce and Bell Pepper

Preparation Time: 15 minutes

Serves: 2

Calories: 120 **Potassium:** 40 mg **Phosphorus:** 45 mg

Ingredients:

10 large shrimp, peeled and deveined

1 cup mixed lettuce leaves, washed and torn

1 red bell pepper, thinly sliced

1 green bell pepper, thinly sliced

2 cloves garlic, minced

1 tablespoon low-sodium soy sauce

1 teaspoon sesame oil

1 teaspoon grated ginger

1 teaspoon olive oil

A pinch of salt and pepper

Method of Preparation:

1. In a small bowl, mix together soy sauce, sesame oil, and grated ginger.
2. Set aside.
3. Heat olive oil in a large skillet over medium heat. Add minced garlic and sauté until fragrant, about 1 minute.

4. Add sliced bell peppers to the skillet and cook until slightly softened, about 3-4 minutes.

5. Push the bell peppers to one side of the skillet and add shrimp to the other side. Cook shrimp until pink and opaque, about 2-3 minutes per side.

6. Pour the soy sauce mixture over the shrimp and bell peppers. Stir to combine and cook for another 1-2 minutes.

7. Add mixed lettuce leaves to the skillet and toss until wilted, about 1 minute. Season with A pinch of salt and pepper.

8. Remove from heat and serve hot.

Stuffed Bell Peppers with Ground Turkey and Diced Bell Pepper

Preparation Time: 40 minutes

Serves: 2

Calories: 200 **Potassium:** 45 mg **Phosphorus:** 40 mg

Ingredients:

2 large bell peppers, halved and seeds removed

½ pound lean ground turkey

1 small onion, finely chopped

1 clove garlic, minced

1 tablespoon olive oil

1 teaspoon dried oregano

1 teaspoon dried basil

A pinch of salt and pepper

Method of Preparation:

1. Preheat the oven to 375°F (190°C).
2. In a skillet, heat olive oil over medium heat.
3. Add chopped onion and minced garlic, sauté until translucent, about 2-3 minutes.
4. Add ground turkey to the skillet and cook until browned, breaking it up with a spoon, about 5-6 minutes.
5. Stir in dried oregano, dried basil, salt, and pepper.
6. Cook for another 2-3 minutes.
7. Spoon the turkey mixture evenly into each bell pepper half.

8. Place the stuffed bell peppers in a baking dish and cover with foil.

9. Bake in the preheated oven for 25-30 minutes, or until the peppers are tender.

10. Remove from the oven and let cool for a few minutes before serving.

POULTRY MAINS

Roasted Chicken with Herbs and Spices

Preparation Time: 35 minutes

Serves: 2

Calories: 250 **Potassium:** 45mg **Phosphorus:** 40mg

Ingredients:

2 boneless, skinless chicken breasts

1 tablespoon olive oil

1 teaspoon dried thyme

1 teaspoon dried rosemary

1 teaspoon dried sage

A pinch of salt and pepper

Method of Preparation:

1. Preheat your oven to 375°F (190°C).
2. In a small bowl, mix together the olive oil, thyme, rosemary, sage, salt, and pepper.
3. Rub the herb mixture evenly over the chicken breasts.
4. Place the chicken breasts in a baking dish.
5. Roast in the preheated oven for 25-30 minutes or until the chicken is cooked through and juices run clear.
6. Serve hot and enjoy!

Grilled Chicken Breast with Bell Pepper

Preparation Time: 20 minutes

Serves: 2

Calories: 230 **Potassium:** 40mg **Phosphorus:** 35mg

Ingredients:

2 boneless, skinless chicken breasts

1 bell pepper, sliced

1 tablespoon olive oil

1 teaspoon garlic powder

A pinch of salt and pepper

Method of Preparation:

1. Preheat your grill to medium-high heat.
2. In a small bowl, mix together the olive oil, garlic powder, salt, and pepper.
3. Brush the olive oil mixture over the chicken breasts and bell pepper slices.
4. Place the chicken breasts and bell pepper slices on the grill.
5. Grill for 6-8 minutes per side, or until the chicken is cooked through and the bell peppers are tender.
6. Remove from the grill and let the chicken rest for a few minutes before serving.
7. Serve hot and enjoy!

Chicken Stir-Fry with Cabbage and Bell Pepper

Preparation Time: 25 minutes

Serves: 2

Calories: 270 **Potassium:** 48mg **Phosphorus:** 45mg

Ingredients:

2 boneless, skinless chicken breasts, thinly sliced

2 cups shredded cabbage

1 bell pepper, sliced

2 tablespoons low-sodium soy sauce

1 tablespoon olive oil

1 teaspoon minced garlic

1 teaspoon grated ginger

A pinch of salt and pepper

Method of Preparation:

1. Heat the olive oil in a large skillet over medium-high heat.

2. Add the minced garlic and grated ginger to the skillet and cook for 1 minute.

3. Add the sliced chicken breasts to the skillet and cook until browned and cooked through.

4. Once the chicken is cooked, add the shredded cabbage and sliced bell pepper to the skillet.

5. Cook for an additional 3-4 minutes, or until the vegetables are tender-crisp.

6. Stir in the low-sodium soy sauce and season with A pinch of salt and pepper.

7. Cook for another 1-2 minutes, then remove from heat.

8. Serve hot and enjoy!

Turkey Meatloaf

Preparation Time: 15 minutes

Serves: 2

Calories: 250 **Potassium:** 30mg **Phosphorus:** 40mg

Ingredients:

1 pound ground turkey (make sure it's low in sodium)

1/2 cup breadcrumbs (use low sodium or homemade breadcrumbs)

1/4 cup finely chopped onion

1/4 cup finely chopped celery

1/4 cup finely chopped carrots

1/4 cup unsweetened applesauce (replace ketchup to lower sugar content)

1 tablespoon Worcestershire sauce (use low sodium)

1 egg

1/2 teaspoon garlic powder

1/2 teaspoon dried thyme

1/2 teaspoon dried parsley

Salt substitute to taste (avoid using regular salt)

Pepper to taste

Method of Preparation:

1. Preheat your oven to 375°F (190°C).

2. In a large mixing bowl, combine the ground turkey, breadcrumbs, chopped onion, celery, carrots, applesauce, Worcestershire sauce, egg, garlic powder, thyme, parsley, salt substitute, and pepper.
3. Mix well until all ingredients are evenly combined.
4. Transfer the mixture into a loaf pan and shape it into a loaf.
5. Bake in the preheated oven for 45-50 minutes, or until the meatloaf is cooked through and reaches an internal temperature of 165°F (74°C).
6. Let the meatloaf rest for a few minutes before slicing and serving.
7. Serve hot and enjoy!

Turkey Burgers

Preparation Time: 20 minutes

Serves: 2

Calories: 220 **Potassium:** 40mg **Phosphorus:** 35mg

Ingredients:

1 pound ground turkey (make sure it's low in sodium)

1/4 cup finely chopped onion

1/4 cup finely chopped green bell pepper

1/4 cup finely chopped mushrooms

1 tablespoon Worcestershire sauce (use low sodium)

1/2 teaspoon garlic powder

1/2 teaspoon dried oregano

Salt substitute to taste (avoid using regular salt)

Pepper to taste

Olive oil (for cooking)

Method of Preparation:

1. In a mixing bowl, combine the ground turkey, chopped onion, green bell pepper, mushrooms, Worcestershire sauce, garlic powder, oregano, salt substitute, and pepper.
2. Mix well until all ingredients are evenly incorporated.
3. Divide the mixture into 4 equal portions and shape each portion into a burger patty.
4. Heat a non-stick skillet or grill pan over medium heat and lightly brush with olive oil.

5. Cook the turkey burgers for about 5-6 minutes on each side, or until they are cooked through and reach an internal temperature of 165°F (74°C).

6. Once cooked, remove the turkey burgers from the skillet and let them rest for a few minutes.

7. Serve the turkey burgers on whole grain buns with your favorite low-sodium condiments and toppings.

8. Enjoy your delicious and healthy turkey burgers!

SEAFOOD MAINS

Seared Scallops

Preparation Time: 10 minutes.

Serves: 2

Calories: 140 **Potassium:** 30mg **Phosphorus:** 35mg **Sodium:** 15mg

Ingredients:

8 large sea scallops

1 tablespoon olive oil

A pinch of salt and pepper

1 tablespoon chopped parsley (optional, for garnish)

Method of Preparation:

1. Pat-dry the scallops with paper towels to remove excess moisture.
2. Heat olive oil in a skillet over medium-high heat.
3. Season scallops with salt and pepper on both sides.
4. Place scallops in the skillet and sear for 2-3 minutes on each side until golden brown and cooked through.
5. Remove from heat and sprinkle with chopped parsley if desired.

Tuna Steak

Preparation Time: 15 minutes.

Serves: 2

Calories: 250 **Potassium:** 45mg **Phosphorus:** 40mg **Sodium:** 18mg

Ingredients:

2 tuna steaks (about 6 ounces each)

1 tablespoon olive oil

1 teaspoon lemon juice

A pinch of salt and pepper

1 teaspoon chopped fresh thyme (optional, for garnish)

Method of Preparation:

1. Preheat grill or grill pan over medium-high heat.
2. Brush tuna steaks with olive oil and lemon juice, then season with salt and pepper.
3. Grill tuna steaks for 3-4 minutes on each side for medium-rare, or longer if desired.
4. Remove from grill and let rest for a few minutes before serving.
5. Garnish with chopped fresh thyme if desired.

Crab Cakes

Preparation Time: 20 minutes.

Serves: 2

Calories: 230 **Potassium:** 40mg **Phosphorus:** 45mg **Sodium:** 18mg

Ingredients:

8 ounces lump crabmeat, drained

1/4 cup almond flour

1 egg, beaten

2 tablespoons mayonnaise (low-sodium)

1 teaspoon Dijon mustard

1 teaspoon Worcestershire sauce (low-sodium)

1 teaspoon Old Bay seasoning

1 tablespoon chopped fresh parsley

1 tablespoon olive oil

Method of Preparation:

1. In a mixing bowl, combine crabmeat, almond flour, egg, mayonnaise, Dijon mustard, Worcestershire sauce, Old Bay seasoning, and chopped parsley.
2. Mix until well combined.
3. Divide the mixture into 4 equal portions and shape each portion into a patty.
4. Heat olive oil in a skillet over medium heat.
5. Cook crab cakes for 3-4 minutes on each side until golden brown and heated through.

6. Serve hot with lemon wedges and tartar sauce if desired.

Lemon Garlic Butter Shrimp

Preparation Time: 20 minutes

Serves: 2

Calories: 230 **Potassium:** 45mg **Phosphorus:** 50mg **Sodium:** 18mg

Ingredients:

1 pound of large shrimp, peeled and deveined

2 tablespoons of unsalted butter

2 cloves of garlic, minced

1 lemon, juiced and zested

A pinch of salt and pepper

1 tablespoon of chopped fresh parsley

1 tablespoon of olive oil

Method of Preparation:

1. Preheat your oven to 400°F (200°C).

2. In a skillet, melt the butter over medium heat.

3. Add the minced garlic and cook for 1-2 minutes until fragrant.

4. Add the shrimp to the skillet and cook for 2-3 minutes until they start to turn pink.

5. Squeeze the lemon juice over the shrimp and sprinkle with lemon zest, salt, and pepper.

6. Cook for an additional 1-2 minutes.

7. Transfer the shrimp to a baking dish and drizzle with olive oil.

8. Bake in the preheated oven for 5-7 minutes until the shrimp are fully cooked.

9. Garnish with chopped parsley before serving.

Baked Halibut

Preparation Time: 25 minutes

Serves: 2 servings

Calories: 290 **Potassium:** 48mg **Phosphorus:** 45mg **Sodium:** 16mg

Ingredients:

2 halibut fillets (6 ounces each)

2 tablespoons of unsalted butter, melted

2 cloves of garlic, minced

1 lemon, sliced

A pinch of salt and pepper

1 tablespoon of chopped fresh parsley

Method of Preparation:

1. Preheat your oven to 400°F (200°C).
2. Place the halibut fillets in a baking dish.
3. Season with salt and pepper.
4. In a small bowl, mix together the melted butter and minced garlic.
5. Pour the mixture over the halibut fillets.
6. Place lemon slices on top of each fillet.
7. Bake in the preheated oven for 12-15 minutes or until the fish is cooked through and flakes easily with a fork.
8. Garnish with chopped parsley before serving.

CONCLUSION

In conclusion, managing CKD stage 3 requires a holistic approach that includes dietary modifications, lifestyle changes, and regular monitoring of kidney function.

Seniors with CKD stage 3 can benefit from following a kidney-friendly diet that is low in sodium, potassium, phosphorus, and protein.

This involves avoiding certain foods and beverages that can worsen kidney function and focusing on fresh, whole foods that are nutrient-dense and gentle on the kidneys.

Additionally, you should stay hydrated, monitor your blood pressure and blood sugar levels, and engage in regular physical activity to improve overall health and manage conditions like diabetes and high blood pressure.

Quitting smoking, limiting alcohol intake, and managing stress are also important aspects of managing CKD stage 3.

Regular monitoring of kidney function through blood tests and working closely with healthcare providers to adjust medications and treatment plans as needed is essential for seniors with CKD stage 3.

By following these recommendations, you can slow the progression of the disease, improve your quality of life, and reduce the risk of complications associated with CKD stage 3.

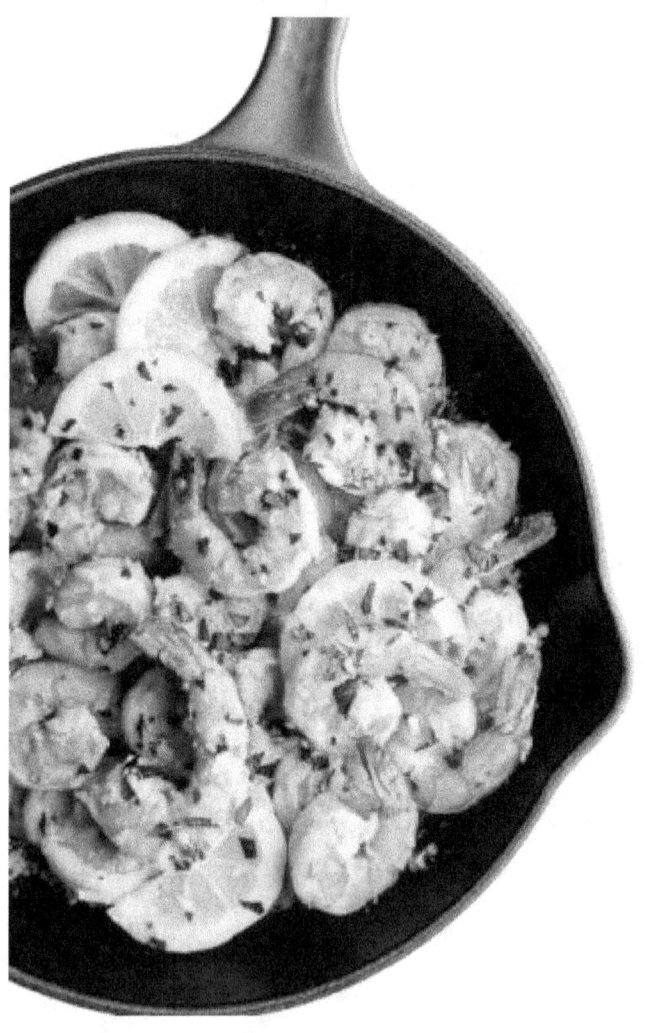

www.ingramcontent.com/pod-product-compliance
Lightning Source LLC
Chambersburg PA
CBHW070435290526
45791CB00005B/1986